The
GROWTH HORMONE
Diet

By Max Rappaport

Table of contents

Overview:

The growth hormone diet, is more than just a diet, it's a lifestyle. This book includes a full guide from the minute you wake up to the minute to you go to sleep. You can choose how much of the advice you implement and how strictly you follow it in order to maximize or minimize your results. The book is broken down into Diet, Exercise, and Supplementation. Using all of these together works synergistically to create the largest growth hormone output.

Growth Hormone is a hormone that creates and regenerates cells. It's what keeps your body growing, staying young, and adapting. If there was a scientific term, which there is, for what you experience physically, mentally, emotionally, and spiritually when you are young that would be growth hormone. If you could put a word for that "feeling" you have when you're a kid, teenager, or growing up, that would be growth hormone. When people say I miss being young or I want to be young again, that's Growth Hormone they're missing. Growth Hormone is more than simply a hormone that makes you grow taller. It affects your entire mood, mind, body, spirit, everything. So, if you miss being young, having a young mind, a young body, and a young spirit, this book is for you. Keep your maturity, keep your experiences, and keep everything else you've worked for but gain back the zestful attitude, and youthful spirit, and take it to a whole new level.

Despite recent claims in the media about the benefits of Growth Hormone Therapy, this book will show you how to do all of that and more, without any synthetic drugs. The only thing you need to do is to monitor is how you eat, and how you exercise, THATS IT! Additional supplements bought at retail stores can be beneficial, but aren't even necessary to achieve optimal results. With this valuable information you can get your body to produce the same, if not more, growth hormone, as when you were young. Although when you're young your body produces more growth hormone, chances are you weren't doing anything special or deliberate to get those results, meaning now that you are following a specific diet and exercise regimen you can produce more growth hormone than you ever have had in your entire life! Now don't worry. When you increase growth hormone NATURALLY, there is no increased risk of cancer, or unexpected height growth. This only comes from synthetic options that are promoted throughout the media. These options are expensive (up to $10,000 a month) and dangerous. My plan on the other hand is free, and will CONTRIBUTE to overall health, not to mention make you feel amazing.

Be warned. This plan might be something you've never done in your entire life. Ever fasted for 12 hours? Be ready for it. Ever gone 1 week without ANY sugar in your diet? Be ready for it. Ever exercised to the point where your muscles are literally on fire, and then gone for another 2 minutes? You will now.

With any kind of reward, there needs to be work put in. There are no free lunches, and this book isn't claiming to be one. The reward you get, being increased Growth Hormone, doesn't come without hard work. It won't be easy, but it will be worth it!

Benefits:

In this section of the book I will explain some of the countless benefits of Growth Hormone, but I will never be able to express through words how wonderful this hormone really is. It will affect everyone differently but there are common changes to be expected. Growth Hormone is like the spark that starts a fire. You never know where the fire will spread to. If growth hormone makes you more attractive, which makes you find the love of your life, which leads to a new home and kids, what started as a simple lifestyle change has resulted in amazing outcomes. If growth hormone increases your mental sharpness, which inspires you to get a new job, in which you quickly become promoted, and use the money to buy a new car, growth hormone was the spark that led to these amazing unpredictable results. So with a such a huge lifestyle change, you can never fully predict the results that will come out of it.

Now on to some actual objective changes you can expect to experience; here is a brief list. I have personally experienced all of these things and more, and so have many others who have followed my advice:

Decreased Body Fat
Increased Muscle
Increased Mental Sharpness
Feeling Younger
More Vibrant Skin
More Energy
Better Mood
Increased Strength
Increased Sex Drive
Increased Endurance
Better Sleep Quality
Increased Excitement Towards Life
Faster Metabolism
Stronger Bones
Healthier and Faster Growing Hair
Overall Increased Attractiveness

Now if that doesn't sound like enough benefits to you, then look on a different planet, because growth hormone is about as good as it gets, and has been described by many to be the "fountain of youth". Now that you're probably excited and eager to figure out how to increase this magical hormone, turn to the next page for brief list of IMMEDIATE things you can do to increase Growth Hormone.

Summary:

In this section of the book I will briefly list things you can do that without question will increase Growth Hormone immediately. Later I will elaborate on how exactly to do these things for the greatest benefit, and why they work.

Fasting
Drinking Water
Exercising
Eliminating Sugar
Losing Fat
Strength Training

Now don't worry. There are many more things you can do to increase growth hormone, and you are not limited to these things. In the majority of this book I will be explaining in detail how to do these and other things, in the most efficient way possible to release the largest amounts of growth hormone. For example with exercise, there is a certain WAY to exercise to release the most growth hormone. With fasting, there are certain times to fast, that will give you the most bang for your buck, and can even work synergistically with certain types of exercise.

Exercise:

Lets start with exercise. Any kind of exercise is going to be beneficial for your health and will likely result in increased growth hormone, but there are certain kinds of exercise that specifically release growth hormone. One thing to understand is that Growth Hormone is released in pulses. These pulses last for about 15-30 minutes where the most Growth Hormone is being released and then gradually declines over the next 2-3 hours. Some things that can cause a pulse in Growth Hormone are intense exercise and eating certain foods. I will elaborate on this briefly. Without overwhelming your brain, Insulin and Growth Hormone are opposite hormones, meaning when one is high the other is low, and they can't coexist at high amounts.

seeking and feeling "the burn" and focus on progressing in a measurable way.

Diet:

Diet! The book after all is called the Growth Hormone "Diet", so fitting, this will be the most in depth section of the book, explaining in detail, what foods to eat, what foods not to eat, when to eat, how many meals, portion size, when to fast, and how to enjoy your favorite foods in a growth hormone friendly matter.

Fasting:

First, lets re-establish fasting. Fasting is one of the most important parts of a Growth Hormone promoting lifestyle. Not only does fasting allow insulin to clear the system, but fasting in itself can actually cause a growth hormone release. People assume they will lose muscle the minute they've gone a few hours without eating. This is not the case. When you fast, growth hormone is released. Growth Hormone is one the most important hormones for building muscle. Muscle will only begin to break after a few full days of continuous fasting. Fasting for up to 24 hours, or even more, will not cause the breakdown of muscle tissue.

Now, for many people, fasting is an uncomfortable state of being, that is to be avoided, or reduced as much as possible. Unfortunately, fasting is one of the fundamental tools in increasing growth hormone. Recommended fasting times are anywhere from 3 hours to an entire day! So, since, you are already in this unpleasant state, assuming you don't enjoy fasting, how can you make the most of your fasting time, and stimulate the most growth hormone during this? Well there are many things you can do. First, as mentioned, before, exercise! Exercise releases growth hormone and is best done in a fasted state. The combination of intense exercise and fasting will cause the body to release huge amounts of growth hormone. Also take any growth hormone increase supplements, which will be mentioned later, during this time. Basically, any activity, done to increase growth hormone, is best done while fasting, because fasting increases growth hormone, and the two done together will work synergistically to give the biggest growth hormone release. Drinking large amounts of water is another action you can take to increase your growth hormone levels. Do this while your fasting! It will speed up your metabolism, help excrete excess chemicals out of your body, and help satisfy your appetite.

Get Lean!:

Another key to focus on in diet, is fat loss. All hormone systems work better when you are leaner or have less body fat. This means while following the growth hormone diet, if you are overweight, another aspect you should add to the diet, is trying to reduce total calories. The ideal body fat to be at, is when you have a relatively flat stomach. This is around 10-20% body fat for males, and 20-30% body fat for females. You don't need to be shredded, and have fully visible abs, although this will help, but at the same time you don't want to have rolls of fat on you. The more fat you carry the higher your resting insulin levels will be and the less growth hormone you will produce throughout the day. In fact being significantly overweight can basically guarantee you that won't be releasing any GH, at all! So the first step you should take in this entire guide, is to get relatively lean, enough so that you don't have huge amounts of fat mass on you. The simple and hard truth is that the average American is way overweight and has too much fat to get the most out of this program.

Although this program in itself WILL help you burn fat, it is best used going from lean to more lean, rather than going from obese to less fat. If you are obese don't obsess over the details in this book, as you will largely be wasting your time, because you will have too much resting insulin for any growth hormone to be released. Your first step should be to get to a reasonable body fat. Although most people find this to be a huge challenge in itself, before you can experience the amazing benefits of growth hormone, you need to be reasonably lean. You would be wasting your time if you bought every supplement I listed and are 35% body fat. You should be 20% or less if you are a male and 30% or less if you are a female. If you are significantly over this body fat percentage your first step should be to reach 20% or 30% body fat, if you are a male or female, respectively. The easiest way to this is simply reduce your calories and increase the amount of exercise you do per week.

What to avoid:

Sometimes increasing growth hormone, is more about what you don't do, than what you do. For example, fasting, is technically the absence of eating. Avoiding any kind of recreational drug would also obviously be beneficial in increasing growth hormone, and overall health. The same goes for avoiding certain foods. Any kind of food that spikes insulin levels, is to be avoided, as this will eliminate growth hormone release for the next 2-3 hours. Any food with a large amount of sugar is a guarantee for an insulin spike. Later I will mention some fruits that can actually increase growth hormone, where the increase would be worth the slight insulin spike, but for the most part, avoid sugar altogether, and don't use eating fruit as an excuse to satisfy your sweet tooth. In addition, starchy vegetables and refined carbs, are examples of food that cause a large insulin spike. These should be avoided too. Here is a simple list of foods to avoid:

-Soda
-Alcohol
-Candy
-Ice Cream
-Large amounts of Fruit
-White Bread
-Pasta
-Smoothies
-Deserts
-Pastries
-Cereal

That might sound like the majority of your diet, but there are many more food options out there that are filling and enjoyable. These foods can be replaced with meat, nuts, vegetables, fruit, and many other options which will be discussed later. This simply represents the majority of foods you find in supermarkets, which unfortunately, largely contain sugar. This is not to say that these foods can never be eaten, but for the most part they should be reduced or eliminated from your diet, and it should be understood that consuming these foods is an execution to any potential growth hormone production for the next 3 hours.

Meal Frequency:

Remember, every time you eat a meal, regardless of the food choice, your body releases insulin, so logically the less meals you eat the less insulin spikes you will have.
For example, if you eat 6 meals a day, you will have 6 insulin spikes, lasting a maximum of 3 hours, which is a total of 18 hours of insulin being present in your body. That takes up more than an entire waking day, meaning you will have insulin in your body the entire day and have no time to produce growth hormone. If you eat one meal per day that spikes insulin for 1.5 hours, because it is a meal low in sugar, for 1.5 hours you will have insulin in your body, and for the other 14.5 hours that you are awake you will have the possibility of a growth hormone release. So ideally, the less meals, the better. Less meals = less insulin spikes = higher growth hormone levels.

Meal Size:

Now, there is a happy medium between meal size and meal frequency. The larger the meal you eat, the larger and longer insulin spike you will produce, meaning eating one 3000 calorie meal a day will produce a large, potential 4 hour insulin spike. A happy medium between meal size and meal frequency would be 2, medium sized meals per day. Now this is not a set rule. I've gotten great results eating 1 large meal per day, and ok results eating 3 small meals per day. Based on my experience I've found eating 1 large meal per day or 2 medium meals per day to give the best results in terms of growth hormone release.

Meal Timing:

Very simply, don't eat right when right when you wake up, and even more importantly, don't eat right before going to bed. The most amount of your growth hormone is released during sleep. Creating a large insulin spike, right before bed, will largely disrupt Growth Hormone production. Eating first thing in the morning gives you no time to fast, which is a large and important tool in this program.

If you are choosing to eat 2 medium meals per day, the best time I would recommend would be 1-2 pm for the first meal and 6-7pm for the second meal. This will cause two medium insulin spikes lasting from 2-4 pm, and 7-9 pm. This means from 8 am-2pm you have no insulin spike and 6 hours of growth hormone release. From 10pm until you wake up, you will have no insulin spike and 10 hours of growth hormone release, for a total of potential 16 hours of growth hormone release.

If you are choosing to eat 1 large meal per day, the best time I would recommend would be right in the middle of the day at 3-4 pm. This will allow a GH release from 8am-3pm and a GH release from 6pm until waking. This will cause of total of 21 hours of potential growth hormone release.

As you can see on paper, 1 large meal per day causes the greatest growth hormone release. This is not an exact science and depends on the foods you eat, your metabolism, and many other factors. If you prefer eating 2 medium meals per day that is a fully suitable option.

Summary:

In conclusion the most optimal combination of meal frequency, size, and timing, for maximum growth hormone release and minimal insulin spikes, would be:

1-2 medium-large meals per day, eaten multiple hours after waking, and multiple hours before resting.

What foods TO eat:

Now onto the good stuff - what you can actually DO to STIMULATE growth hormone. After reading thus far, you should be inspired to have a new view on eating. In terms of increasing growth hormone, it is something to be avoided, as eating causes insulin spikes. Now that you are aware that eating causes insulin spikes, the few times you DO eat per day, should be fully taken advantage of, in terms of food choice. Below are over 10 foods that can be eaten, in confidence, to increase growth hormone, and why the foods work in the way they do:

Whey Protein:

One of the foods that is well regarded for building muscle and loosing fat, is also great for increasing Growth Hormone. Whey protein contains amino acids that stimulate growth hormone. One thing to avoid when buying Whey Protein is a whey protein filled with sugars, artificial sweeteners, and other ingredients. The whey protein should ideally be unsweetened and grass fed. When you check the nutrition facts it should be almost only protein, meaning approximately >20g protein, <2g fat, and under <3g carbs, per serving. If your protein doesn't follow this approximate ratio, it likely has other ingredients.

Watermelon:
Similar to whey protein, watermelon also contains amino acids, specifically, L-Citrulline, which converts to arginine. Arginine has been proven to increase HGH levels.

Coconut Oil:
Although the mechanism is unknown, Coconut oil has been shown to increase HGH levels, in studies, for approximately 60 min after consumption. Coconut Oil is also great for overall health, testosterone production, and has been known to increase metabolism.

Raisins:
As many of the foods listed thus far, raisins also are rich in amino acids, specifically, L-arginine. By this point you might be wondering, why not take amino acid supplementation? That is beneficial and will be talked about later, but eating amino acids in real foods is preferable because they are better absorbed by your body.

Fava Beans:
Fava Beans are some of the best foods on this list for increasing HGH, because they contain a rare ingredient, L-Dopa. L-Dopa is a dopamine precursor and dopamine is correlated with high HGH levels.

Yogurt:
Another food very high in amino acids, specifically L-Glutamine, is yogurt. This leads to increased HGH levels.

Raw Chocolate:

Raw Chocolate is one my favorite foods used to increase growth hormone. Raw Chocolate causes your body to produce more dopamine, which as mentioned before, leads to higher GH levels. Raw Chocolate is also high is tryptophan which causes the your body to produce more Growth Hormone.

Raw Milk:

Raw Milk contains many elements known to increase Growth Hormone such as growth boosting peptides and amino-acids.

Parmesan Cheese:

Similar to raw milk, parmesan cheese also contains growth hormone increasing peptides known to stimulate Growth Hormone in the body.

Goji Berries:

Goji berries are a great tasting berry that contains over 15 amino acids, over 20 minerals, and also are high in L-Arginine and L-Glutamine, which as mentioned before, increased HGH levels.

Almonds:

Almonds, and almost any kind of nuts for that matter, largely stimulate GH production, because they contain L-Arginine.

Grass Fed Beef:

Similar to many others, grass fed beef, is beneficial in Growth Hormone production because it is filled with amino acids, specifically, L-Valine, L-Glutamine, L-Ornithine, and L-Arginine, which are all known to spike Growth Hormone production.

Personal Favorites:

I have no science behind this whatsoever, but from personal experience I've found the most effective foods I listed, for GH production to be: Chocolate, Grass Fed Beef, Fava Beans, Goji Berries, Raisins, and Parmesan.

Conclusion:

There you go. Over 10 of the best foods to consume to actually stimulate your pituitary gland to release growth hormone. Of course you are not limited to these foods, but they should be the stable of your diet, and it is recommended to include at least 2-3 of them per day, for the best results.

There are many foods that are Growth Hormone neutral, meaning they will not lead to increased Growth Hormone OR to decreased Growth Hormone (increased insulin). These can also be the staple of your diet since it is difficult to make a diet out of 12 foods. Some of these GH neutral foods include:

-Chicken (+ other poultry)
-Spinach (+ other green leafy vegetables)
-Broccoli (+ other cruciferous vegetables)
-Salmon (+ other types of fish)
-Blueberries (+ other berries)
-Avocado (+ other foods with healthy fats)
-Olive Oil (+ avocado oil)
-Oats (+ other low glycemic index carbs)
-Almond Butter (+ other nut butters)

Supplements:

As said at the beginning of this guide, there are no short cuts, and no easy ways out, so it should be noted that supplementation is the least effective way to increase Growth Hormone, and Diet and Exercise should be the priority. Nonetheless there are a few supplements that are known to increase GH, and are certainly worth a try.
As said before, although it is not critical, it is best to take these supplements while fasting, for the best results.

Vitamin D:

Vitamin D has more benefits than just Growth Hormone, and should be taken as a health supplement regardless of your GH increasing goals. However, it has been shown in studies, that Vitamin D, through various mechanisms, increases GH production!

Gaba & Melatonin:

If it wasn't made clear before, most of your GH, is produced during sleep. However, with this program, one of the main goals is to create GH pulses during the day. Still, being that most of your GH is produced during sleep, it is very important that you have good amounts of REM (Rapid Eye Movement) sleep, and an overall high quality of sleep. This is where GABA & Melatonin come in. These supplements are known to give better, deeper sleep, and help the subject fall asleep faster. Better deeper sleep = More GH release.

L-Arginine, L-Glutamine, L-Leucine & L-Ornithine:

As mentioned before, all of these amino-acids will lead to greater GH production. Although I personally prefer them when found in foods, and feel they are better absorbed that way, it certainly doesn't hurt to supplement with these amino acids, if you're having trouble getting them in your diet.

Creatine:

One of the most well known supplements for bodybuilding and building muscle, also happens to be great for increased GH output.

Apple Cider Vinegar:

Not technically a supplement, but not really a food either, although Apple Cider Vinegar doesn't directly lead to increased GH production, it helps cleanse your liver and entire body for greater GH production. A cleaner liver, means a better functioning hormone system that can clean out toxins at a faster rate.

Lemon & Water:

Again, although technically not supplements, the combination of lemon and water is great for cleansing the body and increasing GH levels. Drinking large amounts of water is always recommended for overall health and certainly VERY important when increasing GH production, for various reasons. It will aid in flushing out GH lowering toxins in the body, and being hydrated is extremely important in how well the hormone system functions. Lemon is a very alkaline food which helps balance the PH of your body which also helps the hormone system work better. The combination of lemon and water is best recommended to be consumed during fasting. This will create a synergistic effect.

Spirulina:

Spirulina not only helps detoxify the body, but it also has growth increasing algaes in it, that lead to higher GH levels. Spirulina is also great for cleansing the body, and best recommended to be taken when fasting. In fact the combination of Apple Cider Vinegar, Lemon, Water, and Spirulina, taken when fasting, can give the body a super-cleanse and help fully detoxify the body for huge amounts of GH release!

Conclusion:

Although not necessary, supplements can play a large role in your Growth Hormone increasing journey. I believe Diet and Exercise should be the building blocks of your program, and supplements are the icing on the cake.

Putting it all together!

Now that you've read the 3 main sections, on exercise, diet, and supplementation how do you put it all together? How do you combine the strategies used in exercise, diet, and supplementation to make an entire schedule?

In this final section we will be reviewing a few potential schedules that one could follow from the minute they wake up to the minute to go to sleep for increasing Growth Hormone levels.

First lets summarize what we've learned from each section:

Exercise:

Exercise should be done in order to release lactic acid for the greatest GH release. This could mean any lactic acid producing exercise, but the most recommended is weight training with heavy compound movements. Secondly, the exercise should be done when in a fasted state, ideally with 2-3 hours fasted before and after the exercise.

Diet:

Remember, every time you eat a meal, regardless of what that meal is, your insulin levels increase. Insulin is an antagonist hormone to Growth Hormone meaning they can't co-exist in high amounts in the body. This means meal frequency should be as low as possible, ideally 1-2 meals per day. These meals should be low in sugar, and include GH promoting foods such as: Raw Chocolate, Grass Fed Beef, Fava Beans, and Goji Berries (some of my personal favorites).

Supplementation:

Although supplements are not the primary tool used in my plan they can be very effective in increasing Growth Hormone. Every supplement listed should be taken in a fasted state and certain supplements work synergistically such as Lemon, Apple Cider Vinegar, and Spirulina.

Templates:

The last, and potentially most valuable, piece of content in this entire book, can be found on the next 2 pages, where I have laid out 2 full templates from the minute you wake up to the minute you go to sleep, on how you can supercharge your body to create huge amounts of growth hormone.

Option A:

Time	Exercise	Diet	Supplements
8:00 AM		2 cups water	3000 iU Vitamin D
9:00 AM			Super Cleanse: - 2 tbsp Apple Cider Vinegar - 6 spirulina - 2 cups water - 2 tsp lemon juice
10:00 AM			
11:00 AM			
12:00 PM		2 cups water	
1:00 PM			
2:00 PM	Warmup Deadlift (% of 1rm, reps): 25%x5, 40%x3, 60%x2, 75%x1, 80%x5, 65%x15 Front Squat 65% x 10 Barbell Row 75% x 10 3 x Pull Ups - Max Reps		
3:00 PM		2 cups water	Amino Acids w/ 5g creatine
4:00 PM			
5:00 PM		GH Salad: 1.5 lbs Grass Fed Beef w/ parmesan mixed in. 2 cups fava beans on the side	
6:00 PM		2 cups water	
7:00 PM			
8:00 PM			
9:00 PM			
10:00 PM			Gaba 500mg

Option B:

Time	Exercise	Diet	Supplementation
8:00 AM			3000 iU Vitamin D
9:00 AM			
10:00 AM		2 cups water	
11:00 AM			
12:00 PM		GH Trail max: Almonds, Raisins, Raw Chocolate pieces, Goji Berries, dried pineapple	
1:00 PM			
2:00 PM		2 cups water	
3:00 PM	5 min warm up on bicycle 4 x 20 burpees 5 x 15-20 push ups 2 x 10 burpees 2 x 15 dips 2 x 8 chin ups 120 second wall sit 60 second plank 100 bodyweight squat		Amino acids Intra-workout
4:00 PM			
5:00 PM		2 cups water	
6:00 PM		GH Protein Shake: 1 cup raw milk, 2 scoops whey protein, 1 tbsp coconut oil, 1/2 cup yogurt, 2 tbsp cocoa powder, 5mg creatine	
7:00 PM			
8:00 PM		2 cups water	
9:00 PM			
10:00 PM			Melatonin 1mg